Ensuring Equity in a Shared Governance Environment

Marsha Parker

DEDICATION

To my very patient husband who has been endlessly supportive.

.

CONTENTS

1 About Equity

Practicing shared governance is not simply bringing the right people to the table to make decisions. It is also about establishing an environment in which all the players are assured of being treated according to a set of agreed upon principles. The principles of shared governance (SG) include Partnership, Ownership, Accountability and Equity. Each principle must be integrated into your practice, but there is one principle which demonstrates to others around you the level of your commitment. That is the principle of equity. Equity is the most difficult to understand and one of the most important to implement in personal practice as well as team practice. Without the overt signs of equity and the obvious actions of equity there will always be marginalized members of the organization and marginalization kills the culture of shared governance. Equity requires focused attention and purposeful structure to maintain it. The contents of this book are aimed at providing some example methods and structures for supporting equity as well as techniques for instilling and demonstrating equity.

This handbook is written at the request of readers who are dealing with individuals who make work life or shared governance decision making difficult and frustrating. Hopefully, understanding the environment in which equity thrives will help readers understand what is missing in their own organization. The tools and techniques toward the end of the book will help with fixing what is broken. That said, it is extremely difficult to create an environment of equity in cultures which do not value it. However, **do not give up** if you live and work in that kind of place. It is where your influence is needed most to plant the seeds of equity. Revealing practices of inequity in non-confrontational ways does have an impact. More about how to do that later.

This short book also contains some techniques for dealing with those difficult people and the occasional bully in the workplace. It is not an exhaustive work so you may need to find additional resources for deeper study. Check out the references, links and resources included here to give you some places to look. In the meantime, what you find in the contents will give you a starting point or two.

What is equity exactly? It is often confused with equality and while some elements are shared by both, **equality** is more "one person, one vote" as in a democracy while **equity** is "every person has the opportunity to contribute according to their own capacity" which has some similarities to a meritocracy. Equality requires that every person be treated the same. True equity incorporates equality. In some references equity is used to mean equal opportunity. In Shared Governance (SG) environments it is more than that. It is not just that the same doors are open to everyone. In SG each person is valued and their contribution is valued. Status takes a back seat while capability, interest and willingness move people more toward the nexus of decision making.

Here are some characteristics of equity from Dr. Tim Porter-O'Grady in his book *Interdisciplinary Shared Governance*:

Equity

1. Each player's contribution is understood
2. Payment reflects value of contribution to outcomes
3. Role is based on relationship, not status
4. Team defines service roles, relationships, and outcomes
5. Methodology is defined for team conflict and service issues
6. Evaluation assesses team's outcomes and contributions

Porter-O'Grady pg. 54 Exhibit 2-3, 2009

The fifth item in the list is of special note. There must be equitable methods in place for the councils and teams to deal with any type of conflict or service issues. These are "point of service level" issues which are foundational to a culture of equity. All parties must see that equitable processes are uniformly in place and that some are not treated differently because of status. Beyond that, everyone must be willing to speak up if they see it happening. It is common in healthcare that physicians expect special privileges and feel that behaviors are acceptable from them that are not from others. Others on the healthcare team may have become accustomed to that assumption and no longer assume being ordered to do something, which is not a medical order for care, is not okay. Nor do they always think they should have a valued voice in a decision about how care is delivered.

What the doctor says goes, right? Well, not if there is an environment of equity. In your organization does the physician see the people in the unit as his/her staff or as the other team members? Does he ask for opinions? The physician who respects and values the opinion of others on the team is one who will be more successful and have better outcomes for her patients than one who listens to no one and treats others with disdain. You have seen physicians with outstanding technical skills, who are poorly socialized and treat others poorly, have mediocre outcomes whereas a physician who has average skills, but really leads a cohesive team, has excellent outcomes.

When an organization matures in a shared governance approach the members learn to value each other so that a status role does not go unchallenged if there are opposing opinions. The initial adaptation of people in those status roles can be painful and take a while, but once they become true members of the team the things accomplished can be amazing. The team needs all the valuable input to make the best decisions and all players to implement the results of those decisions. Integration of the contributions of each player creates the most value. That means the better the role integration the better the outcomes for patients.

"Equity is not a measure of equality but instead is an indicator of value. Every role has value to the extent that it contributes to the purposes and work of the organization". Porter-O'Grady, pg. 28 2009

Of course, the opposite is also true. The lower the level of integration of the team and the organization, the less value and the less likely high quality outcomes can be attained or sustained. This is why relationships among those at the point of service are the most important and must be healthy, because no one person can deliver an outcome alone.

Since conflict is inevitable, even among the highest functioning teams, clear, agreed methods of dealing with it must be formalized. Just remember that dismissing a person's opinion or input because they have a role of lower "status" does marginalize them in the eyes of other participants as well as in their own self view. If you see someone else do this you must speak up and say, "Hold on a minute, I didn't hear what that person was saying". Or, "Could we please go back to that person, I would like to be clear about what she was saying". Even if it is a misinformed opinion you must show respect of the opinion. That does not mean that an opinion from someone with closer knowledge of the issue will not be weighted more heavily. It will. However, handled appropriately, every respected input will lead to better and better ones in the future. That means higher and higher value from the players overall. It is worth the investment of time and attention.

2 Requirements for a Culture of Equity

People value what they need for themselves and their work as well as what they see is needed for their patients to have good outcomes. That is true for everyone working in a healthcare organization. It isn't just those with clinical licenses who feel the responsibility and who take pride in knowing the people cared for in their organization get the very best of care, accommodations and education. Every employee enjoys feeling as if they are part of something which has important implications for the people of their community. Conversely, no one enjoys working for organizations with bad reputations.

Sustainable cultures require **committed leaders**, supportive **structures** and **processes, integrated roles** and **true valuing of the people and principles** to thrive. They also have to maintain **information flows** about goals and accomplishments back to those who contribute to them. Cultures are complexes of many different things which make up a dynamic, ever changing whole. Those things include knowledge, art, beliefs, morals, laws and bylaws, sports and games, customs, agreed goals and measures and many other things. For that reason, everything you do to build your shared governance organization should be viewed as evolutionary. You can build the perfect structure for the way things are now, but it may need to change in order to keep pace with a changing organization. Keep the doors for suggestion and ideas open and don't consider anything as permanent or meant to last forever. Depending on where your organization is in the development of SG there will be varying growth and maturation. The same is true for where your organization is in its practice of equity. Be willing to adapt to the needs. That may sound like way too much effort, but once you have the foundation in place making adaptions is easier. Here is the thing. What drives the organization to change? The average guy at the point of service must **hear** the goal, **see** the behaviors from leaders and colleagues and **feel** the value of the change. Since every human sees culture from their own perspective the cultural messages must be rich and diverse.

So how do you know where to start?

When speaking of equity think about where the organization is right now. Here are some questions to ask yourself in order to make an assessment:

1. Do I see anyone being marginalized in the work setting or in meetings?
2. Is every person's opinion respected?
3. Do I know the goals we are striving for and where we are in progressing toward them?
4. Am I clear about the value of my role to attaining the goals?
5. Is there a person or persons who have created a "clique" or dominate group which excludes others or is the feeling more inclusive of everyone?
6. If someone from housekeeping went to school and became a nurse would they be treated any differently? Would they be treated differently from any other nurse?
7. Does economic class, religion or race have influence over status of a person? Are biases challenged?
8. Does one's ability to speak English without an accent give a different status?
9. Does everyone automatically defer to the manager or a doctor or is it acceptable to have a discussion with opposing opinions?
10. Are bullies tolerated? How are they managed or not managed? Is there a policy about bullying?
11. Do people make fun of others behind their backs?
12. Do all staff members rotate through various roles for which they are qualified?
13. Are people from all roles invited to participate in decision making? To participate in social gathering?
14. Is everyone helpful to everyone else or only to their friends?

See checklist form at the end of this book or go to www.evergreenauthor.com for a customizable list.

Once you have answered these questions could you give a rough rating of your organization on a scale of 1-10 with one being "Not equitable at all" and 10 being "Perfectly equitable"? Add all the answers up and divide by the number of questions. Most organizations will wind up somewhere in the middle range. Truth be told, most organizations don't pay much attention to anything which is not regulated about equity or equality. Equal opportunity is important, but only measured by a few specific things. If the inspectors might check on access for those in wheelchairs, it will get attention. The same cannot be said for dealing with a bully. Nor will most organizations do anything about pay raises defined by status as opposed to actual contribution or evaluations with poor access to contribution information. Biases can operate just under the surface for a very long time before they are challenged. Yet, these things send very clear messages. Equality is supported by laws while equity lives much closer to the work and must be the job of every player to thrive.

One of the most difficult issues is the technically expert staff person who distains all others with less expertise no matter how hard they work or how much they contribute. These people often align themselves with a particular physician or physician group who then make demands of the organization to the benefit of their "favored expert". These are destructive relationships to equity because they exclude others. This is marginalizing in that those excluded become lower in status and may not be considered for participation in projects, procedures or membership in the same way the favored expert might. This is not to say development of tight, highly expert teams for specialized things like cardiac catheterization isn't appropriate. It is and is very desirable. However, it is how the role is used in relationship to other roles that can be harmful to equity Using technical expertise to develop a powerbase and then working to keep others from that position purposeful inequity.

Even worse are leaders/managers who exhibit "dis-equity" in their behaviors. It is critical that administrators not just verbalize, but also display, a commitment to an environment of equity. Any leader showing a disinterest in rapidly investigating and acting on complaints as well as applying agreed consequences for bullying might as well take out an ad in the local newspaper that they do not support equity. Selective equity is not equity, it is favoritism. Staff are predisposed to assume favoritism is the norm and they will share observed behaviors with each other. So any administration which declares they support an environment of equity and then allows one of their members to act differently can sink the whole campaign. Education of administrators and managers is one of the first steps in establishing an environment of equity. They must obviously and consistently "walk the talk." An example that has obstructed many a shared governance implementation is when a complaint of behavior of a long term manager (one of an "old girls or old boys" group) comes forward and nothing is done about it. Or, if a favored old employee is not required to go through the same training as every other employee, that can send the same message of inequity. On the other hand, everyone can screw up a time or two, correct themselves and still be thought of as an organizational champion for equity. In fact, that example of trying, learning and improving can be inspirational to others.

So what can you do as a staff member when you see a leader behaving in non-supportive ways? Well, if you are incredibly brave you could speak to them directly about their behavior and how it is perceived. Other actions such as journaling the behavior and any spin off behaviors which result creates a picture of how negative actions by a leader can spread and influence others to act the same way. That picture can be brought forward generically as an example you have observed. If anyone asks who it was you can choose to give them the details depending on your fear of retribution. You can choose to take the information to HR informally. HR leaders will then take the information forward as a reminder to administration of the impact of their actions. The council or team working on equity can use the information as they develop their plans for the changes needed in the organization. In other words, there are ways to bring the information forward without stepping in harm's way. Just remember that the leaders are learning too and the person might react very positively once a behavior is pointed out.

For an organization which is evaluated by its members as mid-range or worse by the simple checklist assessment above, major cultural changes will have to be made to achieve a perceived environment of equity. This means a serious organizational education and communication campaign, policies written and implemented, issues identified and fixed and many crucial conversations. Administration members must be, not only advocates, but cheerleaders and demonstrators of the new behaviors.

Processes supporting equity are not limited to taking action against a bully or insisting stakeholders be part of decisions although those are important. Everyday processes have to be reviewed for support of equity. Putting a good SG structure in place is a great step for example, but the current processes have to change for that structure to work. For instance, if a unit based SG council is implemented, but there is no flow of information back to all the players on the unit, or if the information only flows to some and not all, then equity is not supported. If goals are written to apply only to one role then equity is not served. If council information distribution is all by intranet and access is limited then equity is not served. If education is needed to succeed, but only some departments have the budget to support it then equity is not served. There are any number of examples of processes sending the wrong messages. They should be identified and changed.

3 Structuring for Equity

Structures which support equity must be flat with most decision making distributed to the point of service. Decisions in the structure must be made by stakeholders with investment in the outcomes. Shared Governance meets these requirements and is a good structure to move an organization toward an environment of equity. That generally includes basic structures for operating and maintaining a professional practice model. However, unless it is whole systems shared governance, there is the risk that those other than nurses can be marginalized. Great care should be taken to consider all stakeholders in a decision even when the council must reach outside the nursing structure. Additionally, the evaluation of policies and processes for equity cannot be successful without the inclusion of representation of all roles.

Creating a committee or team tasked with reviewing practices and processes which support equity- or don't- is a good structural approach as long as goals reflect evaluation by all the players to determine progress. In other words, does the improvement feel like improvement for everyone or just a particular group? This group should include members across the spectrum. It should not include a person from every unit or department. That would make the group too large to accomplish work. All those areas should be represented on the committee or team though. Representation of a constituency should be a written role with clear expectations of how a representative gathers information from and returns information to those they represent. Do not set this group up if it will not be supported with budget. The work of the members should be valued enough to fund them. That means at least one day a month paid for them to attend the meetings and do the gathering and distributing of information needed.

Valuing the work of those in SG and especially the committee looking to establish a culture of equity means their service is also considered in their evaluations and promotions. Therefore, a method of understanding what they contribute should be established. Self-evaluation is perfectly acceptable as long as some of their constituents also contribute to their evaluations. This is a serious tactical contribution to a strategic goal of creating an environment of equity and should be given the respect of the processes of the organization in the same way the organization would value a very successful improvement team or a clinical team starting up a new service. Their successes should be part of the discussion at the administrative meetings, the subject of success posters by the cafeteria and written up in the newsletter. The medical staff awareness of and participation in the work of these groups is a bellwether of the progress of the organization toward equity.

Other structural issues relate to how old structures are changed. For instance, is there a clinical ladder or general criteria for promotion which includes contributions to shared decision making or process improvement? Are these limited to nurses only? What if a kitchen worker contributes to the committee on equity in substantial and significant ways. For example, one organization which created a Service Council had a member who was an Admitting Clerk who did amazing work interviewing and communicating back to employees all over the organization as well as the patients and families who came through her area. As a result, the organization understood and targeted many service issues such as signage, location of services which were difficult for the elderly to accommodate, inconvenient drop off areas for patients, poor distribution patterns resulting in cold food for some patients, poor documentation of directions to offices and several other service issues. The result was the overall satisfaction scores improved. However, at that time, recognition of that member's contribution was only the thanks of her peers on the committee. There was no structure which allowed the promotion or financial recognition of her efforts because of where she worked and her role. After three years of serving and seeing RNs on the committee earn their service in points for their clinical ladder, she final became discouraged and resigned her membership on the committee. This is obviously not an example of equity and it sent the message that SG (equity) was really only for nurses.

4 Processes Which Support Equity

Any process for work or decision making can support or not support equity. The questions for each process to be evaluated by are:
1. Does this process value each person it effects according to the contribution made or does it vary based on status?
2. Does this process result in inclusion or exclusion of anyone with a part to play in its use or outcomes?

3. Does this process benefit any one group over others in the way it is designed?

These are example criteria. Each organization should determine the appropriate questions to ask about their processes depending on their culture and history. If you are accredited by DNV there is a high level map of the organizations processes in policy which can be a good starting point for the evaluation. Each major process area can be broken down into sub-processes and a systematic review done. What kinds of processes often have equity issues? Any process that crosses department lines or requires interaction of roles with varying status is a good candidate. An example might be transport of patients from one service area to another. Does one area get priority? Is that always appropriate? Who decides? What do patients have to say about it? Do transporters answer to a specific department manager or do they answer to a centralized department?

Also look for processes which may need to be created such as those below:

- Annual assessment by all employees of one or more processes which affect them or their work.
- Application of consequences to those not behaving according to the principles, code of conduct or rules of engagement.
- Requirement for all employees to complete basic education courses regarding SG principles and budget for the classes.
- Easily accessed path to counseling and anger management. Ability for councils to recommend these.

Every organization has a code of conduct, but very few ever assess compliance with the code or take any action when someone behaves outside the expectations. Their behavior is often excused as "having a bad day" or action avoided because someone is afraid of retribution or it is just too difficult to do anything about it. Perhaps that person has learned to preemptively complain to HR about poor treatment by his victims. Unfortunately, this kind of problem could be avoided if an in depth investigation was done of every complaint related to the code of conduct or rules of engagement. This is also the most pregnant moment in developing an environment of equity. The crucial conversation is to address the person's behavior directly and firmly, but without heat.

When they have tried to make you the perpetrator it is the perfect time for a group discussion of what occurred and how everyone might behave in ways that support future optimizing of the work. Smart investigators interview others who might have observed similar behaviors. As soon as there is a good investigation or a meeting to discuss how to improve, the behavior has been revealed and just by that action will be diminished in impact if it is used again.

Imagine the impact on an organization if there were an assessment by every employee of processes which do not support equity and the top three issues were immediately addressed by administration? The reports of those actions would send ripples throughout the organization and would bolster everyone's commitment to similar kinds of actions. Just the awareness of what kinds of things break down equity would have a very positive effect.

The secret to slowly evolving an organization toward more equitable practices is to observe, journal and then reveal, in a generic format, the inequitable practices you have observed. Ask some colleagues if they have observed this kind of behavior. You can leave out names if people are more comfortable. The question many people will ask when you bring up such an issue will be, "What exactly?" and that is the time to give very explicit information about how many times and under what circumstances you have observed it. Hopefully, this will result in some actions being taken. Try to get a specific measure or two agreed among key players that would indicate a change in the behaviors. Even if nothing at all is done everyone will remember that someone observed those behaviors and they will be more cautious about displaying them in future. This process of "revealing" has to be kept in the spirit of observing a behavioral pattern which needs to be improved or observing a broken process which needs to be fixed. While it is always best to directly address a person one on one first, if you see institutionalized behaviors or processes which break down equity then revealing them is a way to influence them to become more positive. Just don't give up. Processes have a way of sliding back into old molds unless someone pays attention to them. Constant, although gentle, attention keeps them aligned with principles.

5 Evaluating for Equity

How employees are evaluated is very indicative of the culture. Old methods of evaluating meant collecting bits and pieces such as complaints of complements and the completion of required tasks or education modules to put together into a once a year discussion. Sometimes the person does a self-evaluation and sometimes there are others selected by the manager or by the person being evaluated who add input in formal or informal ways. The best methods had clear criteria about how a person does in the category of teamwork. Others had questions such as, "Please rate the person regarding their teamwork". Few had explicit behaviors which were to be journaled by evaluators over a quarter, discussed, improvement suggestions made and then reevaluated the next quarter so that there is substantial evidence of the person's pattern at the end of the year.

Have you had an evaluation in which people from other departments had input about how you help achieve seamless transitions for your patients or how you obstruct or facilitate their work in distributing trays, linens or medications? What would be the most equitable evaluations? How are evaluations tied to the SG goals? Do you track your contributions during the year? Who does? How are they measured? It may be that the person who designed, produced and distributed a flyer about a new infection prevention method had more impact on patient outcomes than anyone else that year. Or, maybe it was the result of intensive nursing research done by a team because of higher rates identified last year. In that case it still was a contribution, but part of a larger team effort that made it possible. Without a discussion of what is equitable the evaluation results cannot be used to determine equitable rewards. It may be that an assigned group will have to review all contributions and score their value.

Values should be quantitative as well as qualitative. Actual measures of success including clinical outcomes of patient loads, number of falls per team, number of times the three hour rule for sepsis was met, etc. should be included in the evaluation process. In common structures great evaluations are tough because a very busy manager just doesn't have the time to build the systems needed. In a SG organization managers attentions turns more to creating great support processes and information flows for the teams. Everyone benefits.

No matter the method of evaluation there must be a "real" evaluation of whether the person behaved according to code of conduct and rules of engagement or not. The most frequent evaluation of this sort is a checklist everyone marks very high. It is often a binary option of yes or no and almost meaningless. How can areas for improvement for the individual or the unit be determined with this sort of evaluation? How about if actual gradations of these types of behaviors were used? Or, what if exemplified information was available to the evaluator? What if you had to recommend this person for more education, or to be a role model or mentor or even an instructor? What kind of information would you need for something like that? How would you collect that information? Only if you know up front that you will be this person's evaluator and what things you are expected to observe can you do a good job of reporting. Then it is simply an matter of keeping notes regarding each category.

When people are expected to keep records of observed behaviors everyone becomes more mindful and aware of behavioral interactions and they begin to notice what causes disturbances and negative outcomes. It changes the observer as much as the observed. Thanking those you observe to be excellent exemplars of equity is also very powerful. If you are working at observing those behaviors you will know who to thank.

When a manager realizes that there is a recurring behavior by one or more than one person in the department then an action must be taken. It cannot wait for the evaluation. What can go into the evaluation is a request for feedback from peers about whether this behavior has improved or not. In a zero tolerance environment behaviors cannot be allowed to continue and the consequences must be levied.

Finally, evaluations should evaluate both the individual and the team. Education about team dynamics and characteristics of successful teams is needed so the managers can develop appropriate criteria for evaluation. This is a science in itself and one that get less attention than it should. Again, mature SG gives the manager the time and motive for development of these systems. Empirical outcomes measures development is a core part of the work of the practice and quality councils, is supported by the required nursing research and is inherent in SG as well as Magnet model. The manager then includes these measures in the evaluative systems.

6 Techniques for Instilling Equity

Before the organization has declared the strategy of moving to an environment of equity some problems in that regard have been identified. Common ones such as bullying, inequitable rewards, poor recognition of individual and team efforts require the basic structures, policies (especially a Zero Tolerance policy) and processes are put in place, but there are a three other techniques of value in instilling equity. One is house-wide auditing or assessment by employee teams, the second is something every individual can do once they are educated and aware of the behaviors of equity. That is the personal communication of respect and gratitude for another person's contribution. The ANA booklet *Bullying in the Workplace: Reversing a Culture* talks about "projecting a sense of self value and valuing of others". Even a few people practicing this consistently can spark a positive change in culture for their work area. The third is revealing practices which create inequities in everyday work.

Audits and Assessments

Why would house-wide audits or assessments done by staff lead to equity? It is easy to dismiss the audit findings of a person from the Quality Department. They are simply put into the "they don't know what it's like here" category. That is not as easily done when the auditors are your colleagues and co-workers or when you might be on the next audit team. When the same audit is performed across multiple departments and the findings shared back with those departments the approach is equitable. When findings are significant it indicates some sort of system problem for which resources can be mustered and sensible solutions implemented. That is especially true and effective when some of the staff involved in auditing also assist with solution development. Imagine how much better staff accept findings and changes when they know they may be tasked to perform the audits of the next process. It turns out no one knows how processes really work except those who do them. Managers are often surprised by findings and workers often change processes steps because of changing demands or to accommodate a barrier of some sort. Inequities can develop without the manager even knowing. That is why it is so important to systematically, department by department, go around and ask.

This is a little different from improvement teams in that a major part of all audits should include discussions about behaviors supporting equity regarding the processes and departments audited. The purpose includes the education and awareness of the participants which, over time, creates a base of educated staff advocates. The house-wide assessment of equity can also be a focused review by the council or team assigned to work on equity in the workplace. That approach can have the same effect as long as employees understand that many employees from all areas will be rotating through the council or team.

Projecting Value

Project a sense of value and valuing others is quite powerful. A person feeling secure in their own worth is hard to bully. They also feel more confident about intervening when they observe marginalizing behaviors. People just naturally behave better when they are around a person like this. Not only that, but the person with poor confidence will feel the support of someone respecting them and their contribution and will become stronger for it. A few simple ways to show that kind of respect are:

- Being mindful of the work of others in roles other than your own.
- Recognizing when someone is having a hard time and lending a hand.
- Offering sympathy and truly listening.
- Thanking someone for a special effort even if it wasn't for you.
- Noticing and mentioning how a person's efforts have made your job possible or easier.
- When someone asks a question, stop, face them and pay "true rather than passing" attention

Saying, "I am not comfortable talking about that person in that way" and then changing the subject is a great way to show respect by refusing to gossip or say something negative. While there are often conversations about others going on around you, there are those that are done with the purpose of harming someone's reputation or demeaning their work. It is those conversations which require a quiet redirection. People will soon get the idea. There is something to be said about, "If you aren't feeling it, fake it." When your confidence takes a hit remember it has not touched your value. Value hangs with you whether you are feeling it or not so just recognize you hit a bump you can learn from and keep on projecting value. After all, you are now more experienced having made a mistake or having been criticized. Learn and grow from it, but don't see yourself as having less value. Easy to say and bit harder to do, but think of this; If, in your role, you behave as if you have less value or voice, how does that affect others in your role? Besides, do you really believe anyone criticizing you never made a misstep?

Culture change is a constant. It is always a moving target. Whether the change is positive or negative can be influenced by a few dedicated people who want to quietly demonstrate the behaviors which support equity. When a person is consistently projecting their own personal value and their deep respect for others the bully looks less powerful next to them and will move on to another victim. There is no better way to reveal a bully than to demonstrate opposite behaviors. Additionally, the contrast can move the group to take a similar stance which values the behaviors supporting equity. That is culture change.

Revealing Versus Tattling

In an environment of equity personal accountability, ownership and partnership are active principles. Simply running to someone with more authority to tell them about someone else's poor behavior simply won't fly. On the other hand, those same principles establish some expectations of any practitioner. The way in which broken processes and marginalizing behaviors are revealed are very similar. For a process you would look at how the process is supposed to work, document how it is working or not working now, look at the change in outcome, investigate the reasons it has changed and talk with the people doing the work so see if feeder processes have changed. Often just doing the communicating is enough to reveal the problem and reestablish a working process. For marginalizing behaviors it is similar in that you have to be aware of how inclusive behaviors would look under the circumstances, then you can document how current behaviors are negatively impacting inclusion, investigating why a person exhibits the negative behavior is tricky, but a crucial conversation may show you both something which changes the nature of future interactions. Asking about what dynamics are now feeding this behavior is the same as asking about feeder processes. Awareness of actual versus desired outcomes is just as important for one as the other. People can be so put off by the behavior they cannot see it's repercussions long term. Take the time to think through what happens if marginalizing is condoned. This serious approach to trying to understand is a far cry from tattling. Think of the process like you would an improvement process in the department. Cultural improvement is just as critical since a culture of equity leads to clinical quality and marginalization is a barrier to excellence. If there is a council, committee or team working on developing an environment of equity they are a great resource. You can talk with the group or a representative about what you are observing or experiencing without mentioning names.

Just a side note: tattling is absolutely fine if any type of violence is observed or feared. Safety always comes first.

A Word About Marginalization

It is sad that women, having been marginalized as a group, then use some of the same techniques to move other women to positions of lesser influence or power in their own circles. Marginalization is defined in this book as any behavior or action that cuts off someone else from the mainstream of information, resources, status, influence or power. It is a social issue of disadvantaging someone; not integrating them into the flow of work and decisions is the same as taking away someone's "voice". That is the opposite of what you are trying to do in SG. The scary part about it is that many of us do it without conscious awareness of the message we are sending or it's repercussions.

One of the reasons it may be seen so often in healthcare is that women have become so used to the treatment they don't recognize it as negative. Sometimes the drive to complete a higher level of education comes from someone having felt marginalized and wanting to become a person of power. Then, they use their new power of position to treat others the way they were treated. Some situations are so clear, like the "mean girls" behaviors in the movies, that everyone is aware they are not equitable. The more dangerous behaviors are those that are less overt. Turning ones back to someone who is talking or just not paying attention can effectively marginalize that person – especially if you then divert the attention of the group to yourself. Facial expressions can, over time, begin to move someone to the fringes of influence. While that may give the person who is showing disapproval a feeling of power over the other person, there is a price to pay. Decision making groups and team can polarize with opposing groups just wanting to win against their opponents instead of making evidence based decisions which are best for the patients. Slow, simmering anger and frustration of those marginalized can lead to their withdrawal, avoidance and resignation to their lot. Now you have lost the value of integrated roles and voices which are needed to maximize effectiveness.

Managers are not trained to manage this type of situation or how to reverse the dynamics of individuals trying to create power bases. In fact, most of the time one group will try to gain the support of the manager for their side. If the manager gives signals he or she supports one group then the other group becomes marginalized. If you see this happening it is worth a conversation with the manager. Many times they don't realize what is occurring. Otherwise, a few people working at the point of service who see what is happening a quietly intervene can reverse the impact.

7 Rewarding Equitably

Rewarding efforts in equitable ways is harder than one might think. First, equitable does not mean equal. Payment reflects value of contribution to outcomes. Rewards are the same. In one corporation which had system-wide SG some an individual in the Medical Records department of the clinics made it her personal goal to sign up as many people from the poor neighborhoods to Medicaid as possible. Her purpose was to help these poor families be healthier and she spent many hours of her own time working on this issue so they could get access to healthcare. She helped over a thousand families. The rewards team got contributions from local businesses and surprised this person with a trip, flowers and some nice beauty products. Most of the people in the organization were thrilled and inspired, but there were a few who felt it was not fair that one person got so much and that it should be available to everyone if it were equitable. They demanded this particular rewards program be stopped. What do you think? Was the gift "available" to everyone in that it could have been given to any person going to extraordinary lengths to improve the health of the community? The challenging group felt that anyone who made an extra effort, but did not get a reward would be dis-incentivized. Do you agree? How could you know?

What happened in this case is that the SG council reviewed the process for selecting someone for this kind of reward and felt the criteria should be changed for wider inclusion of possible candidates. The criteria changed and while there was still only one person a year selected, staff who complained felt they had been heard. Some organizations allow staff to nominate other staff for recognition. Those people are then recognized in general staff meetings or receive a modest reward such as a gift certificate for a meal at a local restaurant. Some places do not give large rewards at all. They may have other types of recognition programs in place. The important thing is that staff has a voice in the type of program and how it is implemented.

Keeping pay scales equitable is HR's job, but how someone moves through the scale is often just a matter of longevity. Is that equitable? What is not equitable is when some roles have the option of moving up a career ladder because of contribution to outcomes when others do not. If **all** roles are valued based on contribution and only **some** individuals are evaluated and rewarded based on contribution then there is an element of inequity. This is an item for discussion by the councils. It is a big issue and might require an assigned study team which includes an HR professional.

8 Common Obstacles to Equity

In environments where equity is not a driving principle people are always jockeying for a position of power. The result is often an environment perfect for the practice of bullying. Unfortunately, bullying in healthcare is very common. You may be surprised how many bullying behaviors you routinely tolerate. And tolerance is complicity in the case of bullying. That is why the Joint Commission recommends a zero tolerance stance. You cannot have equity in an environment which tolerates any kind of bullying.

So what exactly is included in the category of bullying? The ANA booklet *Bullying in the Workplace* lists "Common Acts of Bullying" such as:
1. Receiving unwarranted or invalid criticism
2. Being blamed without factual justification
3. Being treated different from the rest of your colleagues
4. Being assigned undesirable work
5. Being gossiped about or being the target of rumors
6. Being yelled or shouted at in a hostile way
7. Being sworn at or verbally abused
8. Being excluded from work related social gatherings
9. Having your phone calls and e-mails constantly ignored
10. Having resources or information withheld that affect your job performance
11. Having impossible deadlines set for you
12. Being denied appointments
13. Being "put down" or humiliated in front of others

Longo/ANA pg. 21, 2012

Does it surprise you how common these types of behavior are in your organization? Additionally, there are acts of intimidation or threat that can be manipulative and hurtful such as work disruptions, stares, sneers, laughter or disdainful looks which are bad from an individual and very hurtful when from a group. Even worse, bullying can escalate when tolerated and become detrimental to the person's ability to get the job done, or even dangerous.

The question for a SG environment is how to recognize these things are happening and then how do two things; intervene immediately and work at implementing culture change that works against them. SG cannot condone these behaviors because they are so contrary to the principles. There is no "in between" that will work. So the steps are:

1. Recognize and document the issue
2. Demand and expect support from leadership and HR including a zero tolerance stance
3. Educate about expectations and zero tolerance
4. Assess one's self and others regarding awareness of what constitutes bullying or marginalizing behaviors
5. Intervene any time these behaviors are observed.

How to go about doing these steps is a bit more complicated. A survey of employees asking how many times in the last month they have observed the behaviors in the ANA list above is one way to start. How you assess should be customized to your culture, but this is a good way to get some documentation about the issue and whether it is localized or across the organization.

At the same time that assessment is being done a small group can be assigned the review of the organization's policies and if they are being used. If there is a No Tolerance policy, a Code of Conduct and Rules of Engagement already then find out if the organization has assessed compliance in the last year. Also find out if there has been action taken for anyone not following the policy, code or rules of engagement. How about action on employee complaints? If none of these things have occurred then the leadership should be invited to respond to the question of whether they feel they have a good environment of equity and what their evidence is to support that belief. Once the assessment/survey is completed and compiled agreement with leadership that action is required will establish the foundation for a campaign for equity.

" Nurses must have the necessary skills with which to address bullying" Longo/ANA pg 16, 2012

This is true, but an environment of equity requires that **all players** be educated about how to recognize and intervene with bullying. Part of that education can be a self-assessment as well. Many of us are so inured to bullying behaviors from our school days and into the adult workplace that we don't even realize we have picked up some of those behaviors. Or we have adopted a stance of avoidance and resignation. Workshops with staff designed to go through these assessments and then learn about solutions are necessary and should be supported with the budget to carry them out.

Solutions and Interventions

It is very difficult to intervene when you have tolerated those behaviors in the past or were even an unknowing perpetrator. Here are a few thoughts about what to do and some scripts to follow when you are a bit flustered. Remember that outshouting a bully or escalating any of their behaviors does not work. It is like biting a dog to teach them not to bite. You have to talk to them and the way you do it is important. Some bullies really do not perceive their behavior is bullying so the first approach is to calmly point out that you feel like you are being bullied and ask them to stop. You can offer to go somewhere private to discuss any issues if you feel safe doing so. If someone else says that to you, just respond that you are sorry and will not behave that way in future. Then really, really think about that situation and if you usually respond that way.

If you see someone else being bullied – especially by more than one person- go stand by the victim offering support. If the victim cannot respond to the bully ask the bully to stop for a moment and try to describe the issue in less aggressive terms. Just say STOP quietly but firmly if you cannot think of anything else and ask the bully to back off for a moment. A safe way to start a script with a bully is to say, "I am feeling threatened or intimidated by the way you are talking with me, hovering over me or cornering me." Or , "I am not comfortable with this conversation. I am happy to set up a time with our manager to discuss the issue." Practicing a script (cognitive rehearsal) is a really good way to help you have a good response without have to take the time to create one. The SG committee or team working on equity may have a person with facilitation skills you can ask to be part of a communication with someone you feel is a bully. Conversation in a safe environment can often lead to deep understanding of each other and establish a different kind of relationship.

Keeping a journal of behaviors is a very smart thing to do – especially in the early days of an equity campaign. Keep the name/s of the perpetrators, the target/victim the date and where it occurred. The journal may reveal there is a systemized practice of some bullying behaviors. Because bullies sometime go to HR in a preemptive way to say they are being harassed when you tell them they are bullying you are armed with evidence to take with you to any investigation meeting.

Risk Factors for Developing Inequity

Whenever the organization or the department is under pressure or in major change the balance of power is threatened and some may feel the need to establish their personal power more strongly. Such times include such circumstances as:
- Moving the unit to a new location or remodeling the unit
- Opening a new unit or hospital
- Implementing new systems
- Major quality failures
- Adding or losing a significant number of employees or more than usual agency temps
- Tragedy or disaster in the organization or the community
- Lack of or gaps in leadership

So if one of the above circumstances exist or is coming up the SG council may need to discuss the possible repercussions in regards to equity. It is important for everyone to know where to go to get help when daily work plus adapting to all the changes gets overwhelming.

9 Key Questions

To achieve equity there must be true investigation. When presented with a situation the council, team or manager must be capable of critically looking at the evidence. Asking the right questions gets better evidence. The principle of equity driving those questions means all aspects are considered and evidence gathered from all parties. It means there are no preliminary assumptions made. So how does one know how to ask the right questions?

Along with the usual "who, what, when, where and how" questions consider the nuance so important in cultures. For instance:

- What are the reasons and drivers for the behaviors?
- What were the phrases or words which could have been

hurtful?

- Is this part of a longstanding conflict?
- What expressions or mannerisms were used? How were they interpreted?
- What was gained by the actions or behaviors?
- Did the environment contribute to the issues?
- Is there significant information omitted?
- Is the information representative of both sides or is it skewed?
- What are the value assumptions which have been made and why?

There is a customizable list of these questions available on the www.evergreenauthor.com website.

These are just a few questions to consider. For help with determining what to ask and how to ask it, the book *Asking the Right Questions* by Browne and Keeley is a good resource. It is helpful to keep in mind that it is rare that there is not any truth to one side or the other. There are reasons why people behave in ways hurtful to another. They may not be aware they are doing it, they are impelled to do it by others or by bad systems, they are not educated about the expectations or the worst case which is they are full of anger. In this last instance caution should be taken to assess the anger level and whether or not there is any threat or danger. Deal with the anger first. Reasoning will not work very well in the face of anger.

10 Conclusion and Encouragements

Above all else, never give up the quest for equity. When you get discouraged just remember that every action for equity leaves an indelible impression that can be a positive force throughout the organization and beyond to other organizations and people's homes. SG is a major change that takes time and effort. Just when things look the most chaotic is just when the model is beginning to take hold. That is also when exemplifying equity is most important. It is the most meaningful thing anyone can do in developing their SG practice. Now you have the structure and the tools to make equity part of your practice. You already work for a healthcare organization so your heart is in the right place. Make equity your quest and your legacy.

11 References, Links and Resources

References

1. Browne, M. and Keeley M. *Asking the Right Questions: A guide to critical thinking,* Tenth Ed., Pearson Education Inc., 2010
2. Isaacs, W. *Dialogue: and the art of thinking together,* Doubleday a division of Random House, New York, 1999.
3. Bohm, D. *On Dialogue,* Routledge Classics, New York, 2008.
4. Patterson, K. Grenny, J. McMillian, R and A. Switzler, *Crucial Conversations: Tools for talking when stakes are high,* McGraw-Hill, New York, 2012.
5. *Bullying in the Workplace: Reversing a culture.* ANA's You Series: Skills for Success, American Nurses Association, Nursebooks.org, 2012.
6. Porter-O'Grady, T., Malloch, K. *Quantum Leadership: Advancing innovation, transforming health care.* Jones and Bartlett learning, 2011.
7. Swihart, D. PhD. *Shared Governance: A Practical Approach to Reshaping Professional Nursing Practice.* HCPro, Inc., Marblehead, MA. 2006

Links

1. *The Advantages of Equity in the Workplace* by Sophie Johnson-Demand Media, http://work.chron.com/advantages-equity-workplace-2635.html, March 5, 2016
2. Shared Governance Forum http://sharedgovernance.org
3. Dr. Tim Porter-O'Grady and Associates http://www.tpogassociates.com/
4. Author website where you can find customizable tools

www.evergreenauthor.com

5. Websites related to bullying in the workplace include:
   a. http://www.nursingworls.org/MainMenuCategories/Workplacesafety
   b. http://www.osha.gov
   c. http://www.cdc.gov/niosh
   d. http://www.workplacebullying.org/

ABOUT THE AUTHOR

Marsha Parker brings over 50 years of healthcare operational management expertise to system-wide process transformations and system installations in complex hospital settings. In nine years of consulting, her leadership in organizational development, change management, and integration has encompassed real-life strategies for process and culture change, including Shared Governance and Clinical Transformation in unionized settings. She was responsible for operational system improvement projects as COO and as an RN and former nursing exec of two major hospital systems. She has also been active in the national and international nursing community as a speaker and author.

She has led implementation of Shared Governance models in several organizations including one corporate wide implementation. Additionally, she has advised on several implementations and consulted for problem resolutions and projects internationally.

Marsha has co-authored *Whole Systems Shared Governance: Architecture for Integration* with Tim Porter-O'Grady and Marilyn Hawkins (1997) and has published several short books in the Shared Governance Practitioner Series. You can find out more about Marsha and her work on her website at www.evergreenauthor.com

.